BUT...
YOU DON'T KNOW
My Story

Women Who Experienced Abortion Share Their Stories

Barbara Conwell Crawford

www.TrueVinePublishing.org

But...You Don't Know My Story
Barbara Conwell Crawford

Published by
True Vine Publishing Co.
810 Dominican Dr. Ste. 103
Nashville, TN 37228
www.TrueVinePublishing.org

Copyright © 2024 by Barbara Conwell Crawford
All rights reserved. No part of this book may be reproduced in any form or by any electronic or mechanical means, including information storage and retrieval or mechanical means without permission in writing from the publisher, except by a reviewer who may quote brief passages in a review.

ISBN: 978-1-962783-32-3 Paperback
ISBN: 978-1-962783-35-4 eBook

Edited by Judy H. Jones

For more information or to reach the author, contact:
Barbara Crawford
P.O. Box 297
Goodlettsville, TN 37070
Barbaracrawford147@gmail.com
www.Perfectlyanointed.com

Printed in the United States of American—First Printing

DEDICATION

This book is dedicated to my mother, Miss Bessie Louise Conwell. Although she went home to be with the Lord on December 2, 2001, her unconditional love and the innumerable sacrifices she made so that I could have a better life will forever be remembered and cherished.

While in my early teens, I presented my mother with this poem:

I haven't a gift or even a card
But I assure you this comes straight from my heart.
You're the best mother a girl ever had
And for me you've been both mom and dad.

There isn't a gift I could give or words I could say
That could ever begin to repay
All the love and kindness you have shown
Through my good times and bad times and when I felt all alone.

So Happy Mother's Day to you, dear Mother
Because for me there will never be another.
I love you; I love you; I love you I do.
This one thing shall forever hold true.

In Loving Memory of My Mother, Bessie Louise Conwell
March 27, 1920 – December 2, 2001

CONTENTS

ACKNOWLEDGMENTS

Grateful acknowledgement is made to:

God, my Creator and Maker; Jesus, my Role Model and Mentor; and the Holy Spirit, my Helper, my Comforter, and my Guide.

The women who openly, honestly, and graciously shared their personal stories for this book.

My editor, Judy H. Jones, whose commitment, tenacity, and extraordinary skills helped make the completion of this project a reality.

The church families responsible for my early spiritual formation – Mt. Calvary Missionary Baptist Church (Herman Street) in Nashville and Payne Chapel African Methodist Episcopal (AME) Church, Nashville, Tennessee.

My Pearl High School English teacher, Mrs. M. R. Walker, who instilled in me a love for writing and creative expression.

My undergraduate alma mater, Tennessee State University, for providing the academic foundation that prepared me for my matriculation at Peabody College of Vanderbilt University.

The faculty and staff of Vanderbilt Divinity School that provided a structured yet self-directed course of study that enabled me to explore my various interests, including human sexuality and abortion.

The churches I pastored that allowed me to "practice" my theology and express my sincere love for God as a servant leader.

Last but not least, my husband, James, along with my children and grandchildren, all of whom continue to provide an abundance of love, support and encouragement.

To God be the Glory!

PREFACE

Abortion continues to be a controversial topic in the United States with pro-life and pro-choice advocates each presenting their arguments in the media and in courts of law. Yet abortion is a subject that few women who are directly affected openly discuss.

What if more women told their stories of why they had or did not have an abortion and shared how their decision affected them emotionally, physically, and spiritually? How might widespread attitudes and behaviors be changed if women felt comfortable talking about abortions? Would their experiences impact the decisions of others?

Families and churches can lead the way in encouraging a love-filled and nonjudgmental dialogue between men and women who have experienced abortion and individuals faced with the decision. Such openness could even lead us to redirect our focus from pro-life versus pro-choice debates to an emphasis on how we can prevent unwanted pregnancies.

This intentionally succinct book recalls the history of abortion legislation in America and provides very informative and astounding statistical data. It also introduces the personal stories of three White women portrayed in an HBO movie and five Black women I interviewed. I found both the information and stories compelling as well as illuminating and sincerely believe you will too!

The lyrics of the song "Life and Favor (You Don't Know My Story)" by John P. Kee (2012) in many ways reflect the feelings of the women portrayed in this book and served as a source of inspiration for me.

Barbara J. Conwell Crawford, Author

CHAPTER 1
INTRODUCTION

Every woman who has had an abortion has a story. These stories reveal personal circumstances, fears, and ultimately the woman's rationale for her decision.

***

During my high school and college years, remaining a virgin was very important to me because of my desire to one day become a nun (The first Black "Baptist" nun!?!). However, following graduation from college, becoming a nun was no longer a goal, and for some reason I decided to engage in my first "real" sexual encounter with a guy I had been seeing on and off during my junior and senior years of college. Although we cared about one another, the words "I love you" were never exchanged. It was during this "one-time only" (and less than five-minute encounter) that I got pregnant.

I had also just been hired for my first teaching position. What was I to do? Would I repeat the cycle started by my mother, an unwed mother? Certainly, there would be no way for me to keep my job as a teacher. (During the 1960s, even married teachers who became pregnant had to take a leave of absence or resign once their pregnancy became obvious, usually after around the third month of pregnancy.)

Would I be "stuck" living in the projects for the rest of my life? So, without telling anyone except my closest friend, who happened to work in the office of a doctor known to perform illegal abortions, I made the decision to have an abortion. Once I discovered I was pregnant, I broke all ties with the young man with whom I had the sexual encounter, so he never knew about the pregnancy or the abortion.

Exactly twenty years to the month following the abortion, I decided to have a tubal ligation. Also, during that time, I had been accepted, on full scholarship, into a doctoral program so getting pregnant was not something I welcomed. And although I had little reason to believe I might have been pregnant, for some reason, I convinced myself that I "could have been" and if so, I had destroyed another life. Propelled into a deep state of depression, unable to eat or sleep, I consulted my regular physician who prescribed Valium to help me relax and, hopefully, sleep.

After having the prescription filled, I contemplated whether or not to take the cute little yellow pill. Would it really help me sleep? Was there a possibility I could become addicted to this prescription drug? Through MUCH prayer, it was at this point that I came to my senses and realized that what I had been experiencing was an attack by the enemy whose goal was to "kill, steal, and destroy" my dreams, my peace of mind, and my life.

Choosing to take the Valium would be a victory for the enemy, but refusing to take even the first pill served as my first step toward healing as well as a victory over his attack. It was also during this ordeal that I repented for the abortion that happened twenty years earlier. I also remember having a "dream" that if, indeed, a baby had been aborted during my tubal ligation, he or she had been "miraculously" transplanted to the womb of another woman who would carry the baby full-term. (With God, ALL THINGS are possible!) At some point, I also had another "dream" in which I saw baby angels flying around in Heaven.

Although these "dreams/revelations" assisted in my healing, for a long time afterwards, I was convinced that a young woman in our church congregation, who had recently married and who "unexpectedly" became pregnant was, indeed, carrying my baby. My name is Amanda, and this is my story.

Until recently, the practice of abortion in America was legal. However, that has not always been the case. America's position on abortion has shifted back and forth since our nation was established. For example, until the mid-1800s abortions were readily available. Although most practitioners had little training, abortions were easily accessible; women could even perform them on themselves. Dorothy McBride (2008) describes the situation this way: "Anybody could and did use all manner of means to end pregnancies; because of the law that reinforced the doctrine that abortions before quickening were not killing a human being but solving a female problem, the regulars [trained physicians] could do nothing about it" (p. 4).

However, due to social and economic developments, more attention was given to standards of the professions, particularly the medical profession. With the formation of the American Medical Association (AMA) in 1847, changes in respect to abortion were demanded based on the claim that there were no fundamental differences between "quick and not quick pregnancies." Doctors also argued that women's lack of knowledge regarding fetal development was the primary reason so many abortions were being performed and believed that it was their responsibility to "remedy this ignorance by declaring that all abortions killed human beings and prohibiting abortion except to save the life of a pregnant woman." In 1859 the AMA enacted a resolution to that effect (McBride, 2008, p. 5).

CHAPTER 2

THE NUMBERS

Two organizations – the Center for Disease Control and Prevention (CDC) and the Guttmacher Institute – try to measure the number of abortions in the United States each year. However, they use different methods and publish different figures. The CDC compiles figures voluntarily reported by the central health agencies of the vast majority of states, whereas the Guttmacher Institute compiles its figures after contacting every known provider of abortions – clinics, hospitals and physicians' offices – in the country. Both CDC and Guttmacher findings are regularly reported by the Pew Research Center, a nonprofit, nonpartisan group that conducts and publishes public opinion polls, demographic research, and social science research (Pew Research Center, 2023).

How prevalent are abortions in the United States? The CDC reported 620,327 legal induced abortions in 2020 (CDC, 2024). Guttmacher's data collection method revealed 930,160 abortions in 2020—the last year the institute's data was published for all 50 states plus the District of Columbia (Pew Research Center, 2024). The discrepancy can be attributed to the methods used by the CDC and Guttmacher to collect data. Not all states require abortion providers to report numbers to the CDC, so Guttmacher statistics are more comprehensive. "It is important to note that these annual estimates are almost certainly an undercount, as they include only those abortions obtained within the formal U.S. health care system" (Guttmacher, 2024).

Based on a 2019 news release by the Guttmacher Institute, nearly "one in four women in the United States (24%) will have an abortion by age 45" (p. 1). Not surprisingly, younger women have the highest incidence of abortions. The CDC reported in 2021 that 57% of abortions were obtained by women in their 20s and 31% by women in their 30s. Abortions among teenagers comprised 8% of abortions, and women over 40 had 4% (Pew, 2024).

Pew Research Center reports have shown, "The annual number of U.S. abortions rose for years after Roe v. Wade legalized the procedure in 1973, generally reaching its highest levels around the late 1980s and early 1990s, according to both the CDC and Guttmacher." Based on data from Guttmacher, more than 1.6 million abortions were recorded in the United States in 1990 (Pew, 2024). The National Right to Life Committee, using data from the CDC and Guttmacher, has estimated that 64,443,118 abortions (See Appendix A) have been performed in the U.S. since 1973 (NRLC, 2023).

Following the peak in U.S. abortions in the 1980s and early 1990s, the annual numbers began to gradually decrease, according to both CDC and Guttmacher data (Pew, 2024). However, the Guttmacher Institute published a report in March 2024 showing that an estimated 1,026,700 abortions occurred in 2023, the year following the reversal of Roe v. Wade. The 2023 number was the most abortions per year in more than a decade, indicating that making abortions illegal does not necessarily reduce their numbers. Interestingly, medication abortions accounted for 63% of that 2023 number, according to Guttmacher (Simmons-Duffin, 2024).

Abortion numbers vary by race and ethnicity (See Appendix B for trends through 2014). The CDC reported in 2021 that among women ages 15 to 44, there were 28.6 abortions per 1,000 for non-Hispanic Black women, 12.3 abortions per 1,000 for Hispanic women, 6.4 abortions per 1,000 for non-Hispanic White women, and 9.2 abortions per 1,000 women of other races or ethnicities in that age range (Pew, 2024). *(Note: Most African American women, I surmise, are unaware that statistically, the rate of abortion for Black women is more than four times greater than that of White women (28.6 compared to 6.4 per 1,000). Is this a statistic that needs to be more widely communicated in the African American community in order to create more awareness and greater concern about the abortion issue as it relates to Black people?)*

According to a Pew Research Center report, for 57% of U.S. women who had induced abortions, it was the first time they had ever had one. For 24%, it was their second abortion; for 11% of women, it was their third; and for 8%, it was their fourth or higher. The vast majority of women who had abortions in 2021 were unmarried (87%), while married women accounted for 13% of abortions (Pew, 2024).

In 2024 the abortion issue continues to generate a great deal of discussion and controversy. Although debate over the issue of abortion in the United States can be traced to the early 1800s, several critical events led to its criminalization in 1821, then to its legalization in 1973, and most recently to a reversal of the 1973 decision by the U.S. Supreme Court.

CHAPTER 3
THE HISTORY

The following events reported by McBride (2008) are key examples of how the abortion issue progressed in America between 1821 and 1973 when abortions once again became legal:

-       In 1821 the Connecticut legislature passed the first abortion statute which made performing abortion by poison after quickening a crime.

-       In 1869, under the leadership of Pope Pius IX, the Roman Catholic Church announced its opposition to contraception and abortion.

-       In 1870 dilation and curettage (D & C) was developed as a method of early abortions.

-       In 1873 Congress enacted the Comstock Act (named after Anthony Comstock of New York who led an anti-obscenity movement) which made it a federal crime to import or sell obscene materials which included information about devices used for contraception and abortion.

- In 1884 Pope Pius IX declared abortion to be against Roman Catholic Doctrine, even to save the life of the mother, because of the church's interpretation that an embryo has a soul from conception.

- In 1916 Margaret Sanger opened the first birth control clinic in America. However, within a few years, she was jailed for violating the Comstock Act.

- In 1942 Dr. Alan Guttmacher called for liberalization of criminal abortion laws at a meeting of the American Birth Control League, which later changed its name to Planned Parenthood Federation of America.

- In 1959 the American Law Institute drafted a model abortion reform statute that allowed doctors to perform abortions under limited circumstances, including: for the health of the mother, a deformed fetus, and pregnancies resulting from rape or incest.

- In 1967 the vacuum aspiration technique for performing abortions (pioneered in China in

1958) became the preferred method for first-trimester abortions (replacing the D & C method).

-        In 1969 The First National Conference on Abortion Laws convened in Chicago, where the Jane Collective, the Abortion Counseling Service of Women's Liberation, was providing illegal abortions. Norma McCorvey was asked to be the plaintiff Jane Roe in a case challenging the constitutionality of Texas' nineteenth century criminal abortion statute.

-        In 1970 Hawaii became the first state to legalize all abortions in the first twenty weeks of pregnancy by repealing its criminal abortion statute.

-        In 1971 a national poll showed that most Americans supported more liberal abortion laws.

-        By 1972 fourteen states had passed abortion reform statutes modeled after the American Law Institute's proposal (pp. 113-121).

On January 22, 1973, the U.S. Supreme Court ruled that states may not prohibit abortion before the third trimester in Roe v. Wade, declaring "the decision between a woman and her doctor regarding abortion to be in the zone of privacy." Since that time, as reported in ABC News' *The History of Abortion Laws in America* (2022) the following events have transpired:

- In 1976 Congress passed the Hyde Amendment, banning the use of Medicaid and other federal funds for abortion.

- In 1981, with the Bellotti v. Baid case, the Supreme Court ruled that pregnant minors can petition the court for permission to have an abortion without parental notification.

- In 1989, with the Webster v. Reproductive Health Services case, the Supreme Court upheld a Missouri law that imposed restrictions on the use of state funds, facilities, and employees in performing, assisting with, or counseling for abortions. This allowed states to legislate in a way that had previously been thought to be illegal under Roe v. Wade.

- On May 26, 1994, President Bill Clinton signed the Freedom of Access to Clinics Act, making it a federal crime to physically obstruct the entrance to a clinic or to use force, the threat of force, or physical obstruction, such as a sit-in, to interfere with, injure, or intimidate clinic workers or women seeking abortions or other reproductive health services.

- In 1995 Congress passed the HR 1833 Bill, also known as the Partial-Birth Abortion Act, which makes it illegal for any doctor to knowingly perform a partial-birth abortion except when necessary to save the mother's life. However, the following year, on April 10, 1996, President Clinton vetoed the Bill, preventing it from becoming a law.

- On August 5, 2002, affirming legal protection to an infant born after a failed attempt to induce abortion, President George W. Bush signed the Born-Alive Infants Protection Act.

- In 2003 the House approved the Partial-Birth Abortion Ban Act, which was signed into law by President George W. Bush on November 5, 2003.

-	In 2016 the Supreme Court made a ruling on the Whole Woman's Health v. Hellerstedt case, dictating that Texas could not place restrictions on abortion services that create an undue burden for women seeking an abortion.

-	In May 2022 a leaked draft opinion by Supreme Court Justice Samuel Alito indicated that the Court would strike down the landmark Roe v. Wade decision, which guaranteed federal constitutional protections for abortion rights.

-	On June 24, 2022, the Supreme Court overturned Roe v. Wade leaving abortion decisions up to states, and no longer a constitutional right.

CHAPTER 4
THE SILENCE

Women who have undergone an abortion experience an array of emotions – from agony to relief and every feeling in between. They struggle with the decision of whether or not to exercise their right to choose (See Appendix C).

In the 1996 Home Box Office (HBO) movie, *If These Walls Could Talk* (which was required viewing for a divinity school ethics class), three different women are challenged by pregnancy during less-than-ideal times in their lives. Claire, a recently widowed nurse becomes pregnant during a one-time sexual encounter with her young brother-in-law during a time when abortions were illegal (1954). The second woman, Barbara, married with four children, becomes pregnant while trying to manage a household and complete her college degree at the same time. Although abortions were legal during this period (1974), she had difficulty trying to decide if this option was the one best for her. The third woman, Chris, a young college student during the nineties when anti-abortion rallies were at their peak (1996), becomes pregnant by a married professor who provides the resources for her to have an abortion.

If These Walls Could Talk assists in generating discussion about the abortion issue and the silence associated with it. For instance, when Claire, one of the movie's main characters, was considering abortion as an alternative to carrying the baby to term, she had no one to talk to regarding her experience so it was necessary that she keep her thoughts and emotions to herself. For many women, as with Claire, there is no one close enough for them to share their innermost thoughts. Perhaps there are no sisters or other close family members for them to talk to. Additionally, due to relocation or other geographical issues, the opportunities for some women to establish close relationships with persons in their church or community are minimal, to say the least. Needless to say, there are numerous reasons why some women have no one to confide in when the need arises.

Again, in the movie, *If These Walls Could Talk*, when Barbara was confronted by her daughter concerning the fact that abortions are now legal and that she could choose whether or not to keep the baby, she avoided engaging in serious conversation with her daughter.

For many women, conversing about controversial issues with members of their own family takes them outside their comfort zone. Others may be reluctant to openly and honestly share their thoughts and feelings due to past experiences or personal baggage. Likewise, some women may choose not to engage in conversations about certain issues out of fear of being judged or looked down upon.

Still again, when Chris, the woman in the third segment of *If These Walls Could Talk* tried to get her best friend and roommate to openly discuss abortion as being the only solution for her, her friend shuts her out and refuses to even entertain the idea of abortion as a viable option. This indicates that some individuals' attitudes on certain topics are so strongly embedded in their thoughts and behaviors because of religious or moral beliefs that it is impossible for them to consider anything different from what they believe. Also, because of limited knowledge or a lack of understanding regarding the issues surrounding abortion, many people do not feel equipped to engage in a conversation about it. Furthermore, there are some individuals who believe that even talking about the issue of abortion causes them to be divinely judged and, thus, they will experience God's wrath.

For some women, talking about personal issues just isn't "their thing" for they have been raised to keep their personal business to themselves. (I can attest to the fact that this is especially true in the African American community.) They have often been told, "It's nobody else's business, so keep it to yourself." For this reason, when a decision has to be made regarding whether to tell or not tell, many women choose the latter.

However, as long as women keep quiet, we run the risk of our voices remaining unheard. And when this happens, we stifle our own healing as well as that of other women who share similar experiences. As a result, individuals contemplating terminating a pregnancy remain ignorant in regard to how other individuals have been impacted by their decision to end a life growing inside of them. Each day, countless women may be exercising their "right to choose" because the stories that might have helped them make a different decision remain untold.

CHAPTER 5
THE EMOTIONS

Although the three women in the movie *If These Walls Could Talk* have a great deal in common with the five women I interviewed for this book (who are given fictitious names), one primary difference is the fact that the three women in the movie are White and the five women I interviewed are Black. As noted earlier, national statistics indicate Black women are four times more likely to have an abortion than White women. Do Black women's stories differ from the stories depicted in the HBO movie? I found strong similarities.

Amanda's story, the story shared in the Introduction to this book, captures the experience of a Black woman who, like Claire in the movie, underwent an abortion during a time in America's history when abortions were illegal. Although their circumstances were different, the emotions that each woman experienced were very similar – agony, guilt, shame, fear, confusion, and desperation. Furthermore, the feeling that no other choice existed – that having an abortion was the only way this problem could be resolved – over-shadowed all other options.

For both Claire and Amanda, the possibility of pain, injury, barrenness, or even death did not surpass their decision to terminate the pregnancy. The only thing that mattered was that they would no longer be pregnant. The single word Amanda used to describe her feelings immediately following the abortion was "relief," and for the next twenty years, she went on with life with seemingly no adverse effects.

For Brenda, the second woman I interviewed, that was not the case. Relief, in no way, describes her abortion experience. Her story follows:

***

I was nineteen years old and in my first year of college. After missing two menstrual periods, my mother informed me that she knew I was pregnant because she had seen no evidence that I had had a cycle. She then proceeded with her usual "speech" that she would give whenever I did something that did not meet her approval.

This time she said, "I don't think you are a bad girl, but I think you are a weak person." At this point my mother took over everything – even making the appointment for the abortion.

The statement that I was weak caused me to shut down and resentment to set in. I blamed my mother as well as the doctor (who happened to be a family friend) for my feelings of anger and emptiness. My mother accompanied me to the doctor's office and when I got back home, I went to bed and cried until there were no tears left to cry. I entered into a deep depression – I did nothing and felt nothing.

I did, however, return to school but had to force myself to study. I also broke things off with my boyfriend and shut him out completely. After about six months of being apart, my boyfriend and I got back together when we attended the funeral of a mutual friend. From this point on, however, my life went downhill. I even managed to get pregnant again.

This time I was careful to "pretend" to have a period because I didn't want my mother to have the same influence as before. When I told my boyfriend that I was pregnant, this time, rather than saying "okay" as he did before when I informed him that I was going to have an abortion, he said that we would get married. So, we got married and the baby was born. Another child was born a few years later, but because of my now husband's physical and emotional abuse, the marriage lasted only eleven years. And although I realized years ago that God had forgiven me for the abortion, it took longer for me to forgive myself.

Facing up to the fact that I was responsible for the decisions I made, I began the process of healing. I stopped blaming my mother as well as stopped feeling resentment toward her. And now, after more than forty years of feeling "dead" and years of on-again and off-again counseling, I have finally experienced "real" healing and know that I can cut myself some slack.

CHAPTER **6**
THE REASONS

In the film, *If These Walls Could Talk*, the reasons the women considered and/or chose to have abortions differed. As reported by Marie Costa (1996) according to a survey of 1,900 abortion patients conducted by the Alan Guttmacher Institute, "the majority of respondents (93 percent) said they had more than one reason for deciding to have an abortion." However, the reason cited most often was that "having a baby would interfere with work, school, or other responsibilities." The second most common reason was not being able to afford the child. Other reasons the women cited include: problems with the relationship, wanting to avoid single parenthood, not mature enough or too young to have a child, and a woman having all the children she wanted or having all grown-up children. Only one percent of the women reported being the victim of rape or incest as a reason for choosing abortion (pp. 148-149).

The reasons the women I interviewed chose to have abortions also differed. Of course, for

Amanda, a primary reason related to the baby's interference with work: In the early 1970s, an unmarried, pregnant woman would not have been allowed to remain in a position as a teacher. However, not wanting to perpetuate the cycle of single parenthood begun by her mother nor wanting to spend the rest of her life living in the projects and raising a child as a single parent also were very strong contributing factors.

In the case of Brenda, however, her reason for having the abortion had to do with the fact that her mother wanted her to have one even though Brenda silently and passively objected. According to the above referenced Costa survey, less than one percent of the respondents chose the influence of a mother or other family member as their reason for choosing abortion (p. 148).

The story shared by Claudia, the third woman I interviewed, sheds light on still another reason some women choose abortion as an option for an unwanted/unplanned pregnancy:

***

I was thirty-one years old, working, and my husband was in the Service. We had just relocated to an army base in another city and were struggling financially. We already had three children, the youngest being only six months old. When I discovered I was pregnant, my husband and I talked about it and with little discussion we both agreed that abortion was the only logical thing to do.

My husband accompanied me to a Planned Parenthood clinic where I viewed a movie and spoke with a doctor. I slept through the procedure and after I awoke, the feeling I experienced was one of relief. As I reflect on the experience, I am glad I made the decision to have the abortion primarily because of the other three children and the difficult time they were having adjusting to their new living arrangements. Many years later, my husband and I finally talked about it, repented, and released it. As far as I can tell, there have been no negative effects.

However, at the time of the abortion, I was not saved. More than likely, under the same circumstances in a different day and time, I would choose a different option. I told no one about my abortion experience except my closest friend who confided in me when she was considering terminating a pregnancy. I actually accompanied her to the same place I had gone.

Another reason the Guttmacher survey revealed that women choose to have an abortion deals with the relationship with the father of the unborn child (Costa, 1996, p. 148). In the film, *If These Walls Could Talk*, Chris chose to terminate the pregnancy because she was in a relationship with a married man who also happened to be one of her professors. Deborah, another of my interviewees, was involved with a married man, and found herself in a similar situation. Her story follows:

***

I was thirty-four years old, working, and involved in relationships with two different men, one single and the other one married. Even though I was using an over-the-counter foam contraceptive, I found myself pregnant. Although I thought the father of the baby was Malcolm, my married friend, I was not a hundred percent cer-

tain. *However, because I knew he had no intention of leaving his wife to marry me and I did not want to become a single parent, I chose to have an abortion. Actually, based on the information I had received, a fetus really wasn't considered a baby so I didn't believe I was doing anything wrong. Because abortion was legal at the time, the procedure was performed in a clinic that catered to women seeking pregnancy options.*

I don't recall any negative effects from having made the choice to terminate the pregnancy and the word that best describes how I felt immediately following the procedure was "relief." It was over. One thing I do remember about the experience that made me somewhat uncomfortable was the fact that I had to sign a death certificate for the unborn child. At some point, I asked God to forgive me and I have forgiven myself, so I never really dwelled on the choice I made. About six months following the abortion, however, I became pregnant again.

This time the father was Paul, the other man I had been seeing. Although we discussed marriage, and even though I still did not want to be a single parent, I did not exert any pressure for us to get married. And because I had already had one abortion, a second one was not even considered. About three months following the birth of the baby, Paul and I were married. We stayed together for ten years before going our separate ways.

Another reason women give for having abortions that falls under the relationship category relates to the father's involvement in some type of illegal activity. In the case of Evelyn, the baby's father was selling drugs and when she became pregnant, she realized she did not want to spend the rest of her life with him. Her story follows:

***

I had a daughter when I was twenty-three. Two years later I got pregnant again, but I did not want to have a second child by the same man who fathered the first one because he was dealing drugs and I felt he was not the right guy. Furthermore, my mother raised all of her daughters to not have children out of wedlock, so I decided to have an abortion. It was in 1990 when abortions were legal that I went to a Planned Parenthood clinic where I first received counseling and then two days later had the actual procedure. What ran through my mind while lying on the table was "God forgive me" because I felt that a child was being killed. The experience was extremely painful – at least ten times more painful than regular menstrual cramps. After it was over, the friend who accompanied me and I discussed another friend who used abortion as a means of birth control. We could not believe that she had undergone at least thirteen abortions.

At this point in life, I have no regrets because I feel certain it was the right decision for me to have made during that phase of my life. So, without a doubt, "relief" is the one word I would use to describe the experience. Consciously, I experienced no ill effects although after I got married and my first pregnancy resulted in a miscarriage, I thought that it might have been in some way connected to the abortion. I feel that I have had a great life thus far; however, because now I am more mature than I was twenty-five years ago, I would probably make some different life choices.

Again, throughout history, for a variety of reasons, abortions have been experienced by women of different ages, ethnicities, and socioeconomic levels. Furthermore, these women have encountered an array of emotions and effects. Even the women I interviewed who indicated that they were relieved once the abortion was over, also indicated that the issue resurfaced at some point later in life.

Chapter 7
CONCLUSION

One thing all five of the women I interviewed have in common is that prior to their interview with me, none of them had discussed their abortion with anyone different from the person they confided in when it happened many years earlier. As previously stated, women who have experienced abortion have a tendency to remain silent regarding the issue. Therefore, we must now stake the claim that talking about our lived realities is essential. The weightier matter of saying "But you don't know my story" must be considered more deeply in terms of posing basic questions about when, where, and how to best voice our experiences and feelings.

It is my contention that female-bodied persons who have experienced abortion must become willing to talk about their experiences. In other words, *saying* "But you don't know my story" and then *telling* that story becomes crucial.

The following recommendations are presented in hopes that they will lead to desired and viable solutions.

First of all, women who have experienced abortion (as well as women who have not) must become more knowledgeable regarding the topic and the varied and complicated issues surrounding it. While seeking out women interested in sharing their stories, I discovered that many of the individuals I spoke to were unclear regarding their stand on abortion – they were unsure whether their position was one of pro-life or pro-choice. Women must, therefore, make a conscious effort to acquire the knowledge necessary to determine where they stand on the issue so that they will feel comfortable engaging in conversations with one another as well as with individuals outside of their gender and culture.

Secondly, after acquiring the knowledge, women must then find ways to share it with others. Again, abortion is not an issue openly discussed in most settings. However, in order for women who have experienced abortion to openly share their experiences with others, they must first rid themselves of the guilt and shame attached to that experience. The saying "Confession is good for the soul" certainly applies in regard to abortion. Furthermore, James 5:16 (New International Version) clearly says, "Confess your sins to one another and pray for one another that you may be healed." Once loosened from those dormant emotions, women are better able to move forward and, in the process, help others do the same.

Certainly, a good place to begin abortion dialogue would be in the church. Conversations within church settings such as Bible Studies and Prayer Groups would be beneficial to the Body of Christ. Rather than focusing so much time and attention on outward appearance, perhaps the time has arrived for women and men to think more deeply and converse more openly about the issues that affect our inward beauty. The moral choices related to abortion certainly qualify for such dialogue.

Likewise, finding ways to incorporate human sexuality into sermons as a means of addressing the behaviors that make abortion decisions necessary in the first place would certainly provide opportunities for church members to openly and honestly discuss topics such as fornication and adultery. Even though embarrassment and discomfort sometimes accompany discussions that deal with sexuality, the inviting and non-judgmental atmosphere prayerfully espoused by most churches makes them the ideal setting for such discussions to occur.

Furthermore, involving outside parties trained in leading discussions on topics related to human sexuality and its numerous facets would be a good way to generate conversations about abortion with both young and old alike. Inviting women (and men) who have experienced abortion to share their stories would certainly generate some much-needed discussion.

Thirdly, as mothers, grandmothers, sisters, aunts, cousins, and friends, it is certainly reasonable to assume that women can have a positive influence on the young women that follow behind us. When our younger relatives and friends ask us to share our lived experiences, rather than putting them off or making it appear that such discussions are off limits, women must welcome the opportunity to engage in conversation with them and then openly and honestly share their thoughts and feelings.

Women also must be willing to initiate dialogue about various issues in an effort to generate interest in topics they might otherwise not consider discussing. The motive, however, must not be to persuade our young cohorts to think as we think, but rather for them to think for themselves.

Today our youth are greatly influenced by what they see and hear in the media. Perhaps the voices of the women these young people encounter in their own homes, churches, and communities can counteract or overshadow the less than positive voices and images portrayed through the media. Perhaps our young girls will begin to gravitate more toward us -- as up-close, caring, and concerned role models and mentors -- rather than toward the distant images that constantly and aggressively invade their social spaces.

Although the individuals portrayed in media may not be discussing the issue of abortion, they are, no doubt, promoting the sexual behaviors that eventually lead to decisions surrounding abortion. Interestingly, these "celebrities" frequently self-report about everything imaginable – drug and alcohol abuse, unfaithfulness in their marriages, weight loss, eating disorders, etc. Oftentimes, they rally for or against these issues and causes. However, rarely (if at all) do any of them speak out for or against abortion.

Is it possible that celebrities speaking out about their abortion experience, especially the ones that experienced lingering emotional or spiritual distress, would affect the way society views abortion? Likewise, if more "regular" women spoke up about the negative long-term effects of their abortion experiences, is it possible that more women might choose another option?

Theoretically, politically, morally, and philosophically, abortion remains a highly discussed and debated subject. But where are these discussions and debates taking place? Are the individuals involved in these conversations the ones with the ability to effect changes in attitudes and behaviors? Are mothers talking to daughters? Are fathers talking to sons? Are friends talking to friends? Are church leaders talking to their members? Are persons who have experienced an abortion talking to those individuals contemplating having one?

It might appear that almost everyone has his or her mind made up concerning abortion and, therefore, no further discussion is needed. However, based on conversations with family members, friends, colleagues, and church members, many people are still unsure where they stand on the issue. Furthermore, based on past moral issues (slavery, women's voting rights, child labor, etc.) which were hotly debated and are now objects of widespread consensus, change is possible, even with regard to the issue of abortion (Kaczor, 2011, p. 2).

Marie Costa, author of *Abortion: Contemporary World Issues (1996)*, begins her book with the following statement: "Abortion, a word once rarely spoken out loud, has over the last three decades become synonymous with controversy and conflict. Many of those involved seem to feel that they are at war with an enemy that strikes at the heart of their values and beliefs, at the whole order by which they organize their lives" (p. xiii).

Although a source of controversy throughout history and a common experience for women in the United States, today the abortion issue appears most often fought in courtrooms and the legislature. Mary Cunningham Agee, founder of the Nurturing Network says, "Both the 'pro-life' and 'pro-choice' movements—characterized most often by their emotionally-charged legislative battles, rhetorical debates and judgmental protests – often overlook the imminent needs of the woman about whom they are arguing" (Costa, 1996, p. xv).

Interestingly, at one point in history, not only was the word abortion rarely spoken out loud, it was and continues to be rarely spoken at all among the people that are most directly affected. This, of course, leads to my original point: Stories regarding women's abortion experiences are not being heard primarily because they are not being told. As a result, individuals faced with the decision to choose an abortion or some other alternative oftentimes make decisions without the benefit of hearing these stories. But once families, churches, and even schools begin to more openly discuss the issue of abortion, then and only then will attitudes and behaviors change. Only then will a drastic reduction be made in the number of abortions performed each year. Only then will the guilt and shame suffered by so many individuals, males and females, who later regret their decision, be squelched.

Perhaps the time has come for us to redirect our focus from the pro-life/pro-choice debates and begin focusing our attention on an area of discussion that actually gets to the core of the problem – the *prevention* of unwanted pregnancies. Prevention can occur not only through the use of appropriate birth control measures, but also by digging deep into the moral fiber of our society and making some much needed changes, especially in regard to issues surrounding human sexuality. Although other societal ills such as mass shootings and various other forms of violence bombard our nation and communities, redirecting our focus to include the prevention of unwanted pregnancies is a great place to start. When unwanted pregnancies are prevented, the need for abortions diminishes.

I am truly grateful for the opportunity to share my story (one of the five women interviewed) as well as the stories of the other women included in this book and pray that everyone who reads our stories will be inspired to share their own story. By doing so, it is my hope (and belief) that countless others will benefit and be blessed in the same way I have been.

As a woman who has experienced abortion, I no longer have the tendency to remain silent regarding the issue by keeping my experience to myself, for I am no longer fearful of the judgmental attitudes exhibited by others. Likewise, due to different manifestations of shame, as a female-bodied person with children as well as grandchildren, I no longer have the tendency to inhibit possibilities of healing by avoiding those who ask difficult questions.

Lastly, no longer am I refusing to speak out about my lived reality due to a fear of appearing "less than." Nor will I deflect questions regarding my stand (or, perhaps, dual stand) on the pro-life/pro-choice debate, but instead espouse my newly created position of *"pro-prevention."*

The song "Life and Favor (You Don't Know My Story)" (Kee, 2012) inspired me because it speaks of pain, fear, shame, and judgment and embodies the experiences of so many women who have had an abortion. But most important, the song also speaks of deliverance and the promise that regardless of our experiences, God can use us through the telling of our stories. To God be the Glory!

REFERENCES

Babic, I. & Richardson, E. *Abortion in America: A Visual Timeline, The History of Abortion*

Laws in America. (2022, June 24). ABC News. Retrieved from https://abcnews.go.com/Politics/abortion-america-visual-timelinestory

Centers for Disease Control and Prevention (CDC). (2024). *CDC's Abortion Surveillance System.* Retrieved from https://www.cdc.gov/reproductivehealth/data_ stats/abortion.htm

Costa, M. (1996). *Abortion: A Reference Handbook.* Santa Barbara, CA: ABC-CLIO, Inc.

Guttmacher Institute. (2019, September). *Induced Abortion in the United States.* Retrieved from https://www.guttmacher.org/fact-sheet/induced-abortion-united-states

Guttmacher Institute. (2024, March). *Despite Bans, Number of Abortions in the United States*

Increased in 2023. Retrieved from https://www.guttmacher.org/2024/03/despite-bans-number-abortions-united-states-increased-2023

Kaczor, C. (2011). *The Ethics of Abortion: Women's Rights, Human Life, and the Question of Justice.* New York, NY: Routledge.

Kee, J. P. (2012). *Life and Favor (You Don't Know My Story).* Available on Spotify.com https://open.spotify.com/track/0Z2DaKiwLWfTuItxHWFTsR

McBride, D. (2008). *Abortion in the United States.* Santa Barbara, CA: ABC-CLIO, Inc.

National Right to Life Committee. (2023, January 23). *The State of Abortion in the United-States, 2023.* Retrieved from https://www.nrlc.org/uploads/factsheets/23StatsFS.pdf

Pew Research Center. (2024, March 25). *What the data says about abortion in the U.S.*

Retrieved from https://www.pewresearch.org/short-reads/2024/03/25/what-the-data-says-about-abortion-in-the-us/

Savoca, N. and Cher (Directors). (1996). *If These Walls Could Talk.* [Television film]. HBO NYC Productions.

Simmons-Duffin, S. (2024, March 19). *Despite bans in some states, more than a million abortions were provided in 2023* [Audio Transcript]. Retrieved from https://www.npr.org/sections/health-shots/2024/03/19/1238293143/abortion-data-how-many-us-2023

APPENDIX

Reported Annual Abortions

	Guttmacher	CDC
1973	744,610	615,831
1974	898,570	763,476
1975	1,034,170	854,853
1976	1,179,300	988,267
1977	1,316,700	1,079,430
1978	1,409,600	1,157,776
1979	1,497,670	1,251,921
1980	1,553,890	1,297,606
1981	1,577,340	1,300,760
1982	1,573,920	1,303,980
1983	1,575,000	1,268,987
1984	1,577,180	1,333,521
1985	1,588,550	1,328,570
1986	1,574,000	1,328,112
1987	1,559,110	1,353,671
1988	1,590,750	1,371,285
1989	1,566,900	1,396,658
1990	1,608,600	1,429,247
1991	1,556,510	1,388,937
1992	1,528,930	1,359,146
1993	1,495,000	1,330,414
1994	1,423,000	1,267,415
1995	1,359,400	1,210,883
1996	1,360,160	1,225,937
1997	1,335,000	1,186,039
1998	1,319,000	884,273*
1999	1,314,800	861,789*
2000	1,312,990	857,475*
2001	1,291,000	853,485*
2002	1,269,000	854,122*
2003	1,250,000	848,163*
2004	1,222,100	839,226*
2005	1,206,200	820,151*
2006	1,242,200	852,385*
2007	1,209,640	827,609*
2008	1,212,350	825,564*
2009	1,151,600	789,217*
2010	1,102,670	765,651*
2011	1,058,490	730,322*
2012	1,011,000	699,202*
2013	958,700	664,435*
2014	926,190	652,639*
2015	899,500	638,169*
2016	874,100	623,471*
2017	862,320	612,719*
2018	885,800	619,591*
2019	916,640	629,898*
2020	930,160	620,327*
2021	930,160 §	
2022	900,414 §	

*Excludes NH, CA and often at least one other state.

§ NRLC projection for calculation

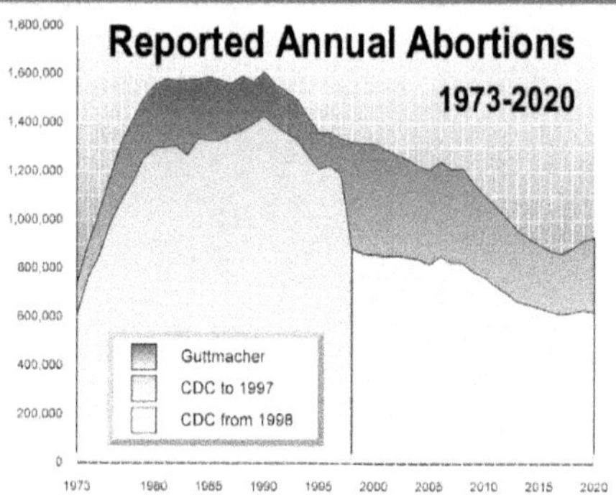

ABORTION STATISTICS

United States Data and Trends

There are two basic sources on abortion data in the U.S.:

- The U.S. Centers for Disease Control (CDC) publishes yearly, but relies on voluntary reports from state health departments (and New York City, Washington, D.C.). It has been missing data from California, New Hampshire, and at least one other state since 1998.
- The Guttmacher Institute (GI) contacts abortion clinics directly for data but does not always survey every year.
- Because it surveys clinics directly and includes data from all fifty states, most re-searchers believe Guttmacher's numbers to be more reliable, though Guttmacher still believes it may miss some abortions.

While both Guttmacher and the CDC show big drops over the last 30 years, recent years show increases.

- Total abortions dropped 29.8% from 1998 to 2020 with the CDC, and fell 42.2% from 1990 to 2020 with GI.
- The **abortion rate** for 2020 for GI was 14.4 abortions for every 1,000 women of re-productive age (15-44), less than half that of the high of 29.3 in 1981. While up since 2017 (13.5), it is still lower than when abortion was legalized in the U.S. in 1973 (16.3).
- GI says there were 20.6 abortions for every 100 pregnancies ending in live birth or abortion in 2020, up from 18.3 in 2016, the lowest **abortion ratio** since 1972.
- GI says that abortion "providers" rose slightly to 1,603 in 2020 from 1,587 in 2017. The high was 2,918 in 1982.
- According to the GI, more than half (53%) of abortions were done with chemical abortifacients like mifepristone in 2020. It had been just 16.4% as recently as 2008.
- In June 2022, *Dobbs* overturned *Roe*, activating "trigger laws" in some states offering the unborn full protection or otherwise limiting abortion. Many clinics closed, but some women went to other states or ordered abortion pills online.

The Consequences of *Roe v. Wade*

64,443,118

Total abortions since 1973

Based on numbers reported by the Guttmacher Institute 1973-2020, with 3% added for GI estimated possible 3-5% undercount for 1973-2014. Additional 12,000 per year for 2015-2017 for abortions from "providers" GI says it may have missed in 2015-2017 counts. 2022 estimate projects drops from states with trigger laws since *Dobbs*. 01/23

GUTTMACHER INSTITUTE

Abortion rates continue to vary
by race and ethnicity

Lack of access to health insurance and health care plays a
role, as do racism and discrimination

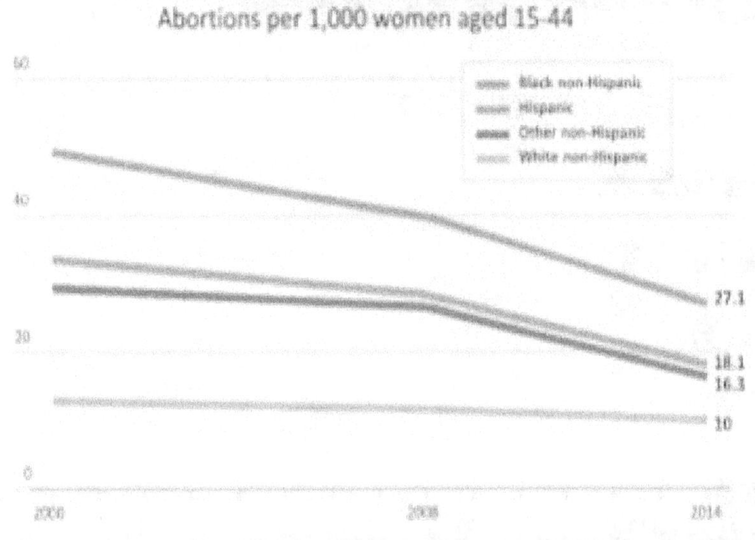

gu.tt/Abortion2014   ©2017

https://www.guttmacher.org/infographic/2017/abortion-rates-race-and-ethnicity

Appendix C Reasons for Abortions

Reasons U.S. Women Have Abortions

Most Important Reasons Cited

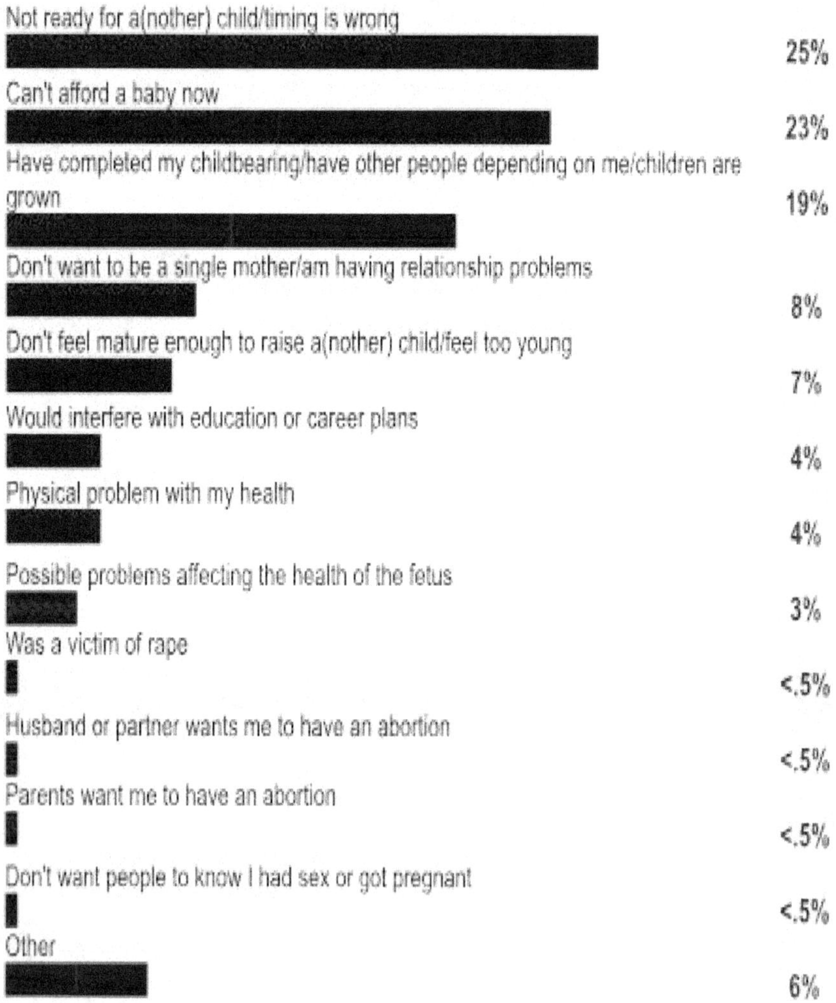
Not ready for a(nother) child/timing is wrong 25%
Can't afford a baby now 23%
Have completed my childbearing/have other people depending on me/children are grown 19%
Don't want to be a single mother/am having relationship problems 8%
Don't feel mature enough to raise a(nother) child/feel too young 7%
Would interfere with education or career plans 4%
Physical problem with my health 4%
Possible problems affecting the health of the fetus 3%
Was a victim of rape <.5%
Husband or partner wants me to have an abortion <.5%
Parents want me to have an abortion <.5%
Don't want people to know I had sex or got pregnant <.5%
Other 6%

Note: This survey of 957 women having an abortion was first published by Guttmacher Institute in September 2005. Data retrieved from https://www.guttmacher.org/sites/default/files/pdfs/tables/370305/3711005t3.pdf

APPENDIX D

But...*You Don't Know My Story*

Interview Questions

1. How old were you when the abortion happened?

2. What was your situation at the time? (Student, working, in a relationship, etc.)

3. Describe in your own words the circumstances surrounding your decision to have an abortion.

4. Where did the abortion take place?

5. Were there other people around you or with you when the abortion took place?

6. Did you understand what was happening to you?

7. Do you remember what you were thinking or feeling at the time?

8. What happened after the abortion?

9. What ONE word BEST describes how you felt immediately following the abortion? (Guilt, shame, agony, embarrassment, pain (physical or emotional), relief, etc.

10. What (if any) negative effects have you had

since the abortion?

11. At the time, did you tell anyone how you were feeling or what was happening to you? Did they help you? Did you ever seek counseling? Have you ever shared your abortion experience with family members or friends?

12. What has your life been like since the abortion?

ABOUT THE AUTHOR

Reverend Barbara J. Conwell Crawford, Ed. D., M. Div.

Dr. Barbara Conwell Crawford is a retired pastor and educator living in Goodlettsville, TN. She credits her favorite scripture, Romans 8:28, as inspiration for her life's work, because she *truly* loves the Lord, believes she has been called according to *His* purpose, and that all things *always* work together for the good!

Dr. Crawford served as Pastor of St. Luke African Methodist Episcopal (AME) Church, Gallatin, Tennessee, for five years prior to her retirement in October 2023. Previously, the Nashville native served as pastor of St. Luke AME Church in Nashville, Tennessee, and St. Paul AME Church in Woodburn, Kentucky. An ordained Elder in the African Methodist Episcopal Church since 1996, Dr. Crawford faithfully served as Assistant Pastor of Payne Chapel AME Church, Nashville, for more than 20 years under the pastorate of Rev. Sidney F. Bryant.

Dr. Crawford retired from the Metropolitan

Nashville Public School System in 2007. During her 37 years with Metro Schools, she served as a teacher, reading specialist, and principal. She began her teaching career as one of the first African American teachers assigned to a previously all-White school. Under her leadership as principal of Wharton Middle School, Nashville's middle school arts magnet program was established.

A life-long learner, Dr. Crawford received a Bachelor of Science degree in Elementary Education from Tennessee (A&I) State University (1969), a Master's Degree in Reading from Middle Tennessee State University (1976), a +30 Endorsement in Administration and Supervision from Tennessee State University (1986), and a Doctor of Education degree from Peabody College of Vanderbilt University (1991). She received a Master of Divinity degree from Vanderbilt University in 2014.

Dr. Crawford has been recognized for her service to children, the church, and the community. Her honors include: National Council of Christians and Jews Brotherhood-Sisterhood Educator of the Year Award, HCA Teacher

Award, Frist Principal Award, and UPN Nashville Principal of the Month. In 2017 she was recognized for having completed the Goodlettsville Leadership Academy. Dr. Crawford is a member of Delta Sigma Theta Sorority, Inc.

An itinerant elder serving in the AME Tennessee Conference, Dr. Crawford was recognized in 2018 by the Conference's Lay Organization as a "Pastor of the Year." She has served as a member of the Tennessee Conference Board of Examiners, chair of the Tennessee Conference Christian Education Committee, and Secretary and past President of the Gallatin United Ministerial Alliance.

Dr. Crawford and her husband, James, celebrated their 50th wedding anniversary June 9, 2023. They are the proud parents of two sons, Rev. Marlan E. Crawford and Michael A. Crawford, Sr.; daughter-in-love, Sarita; and three grandchildren, Michael Jr., Jordan Jeanee, and Mason.

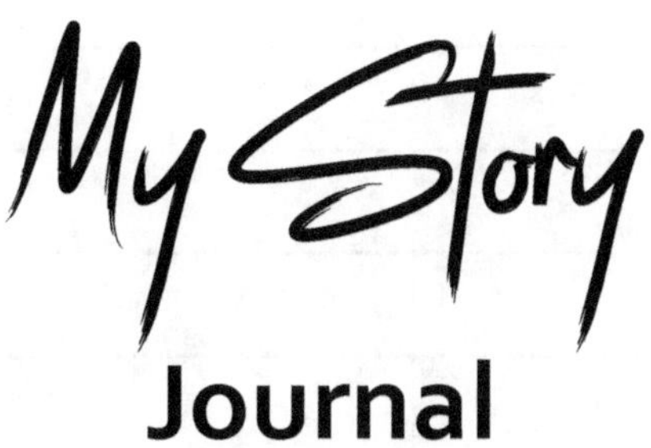

Journal

Tell Your Story

www.ingramcontent.com/pod-product-compliance
Lightning Source LLC
Chambersburg PA
CBHW050012070726
47598CB00014B/754